Yoga For Beginners

30 Essential Yoga Poses to Transform Your Mind, Body & Spirit

Learn Yoga in Just 10 Minutes a Day

Olivia Summers

Published in The USA by:

Success Life Publishing

125 Thomas Burke Dr.

Hillsborough, NC 27278

Copyright © 2015 by Olivia Summers

ISBN-10: 1511682574

Table of Contents

Introduction

Thank you so much for purchasing my book "Yoga For Beginners." My name is Olivia Summers and I'm a Certified Yoga Teacher and for the duration of this book I'm going to personally be by your side coaching you along for the next 30 days.

One thing I'd like to point out, though, is that the time frame I use is just a starting off point. You can spend as much time as you'd like on each pose. In the book I suggest just 10 minutes as you're starting point and that's perfectly acceptable. You will gain a much better perspective of yoga just by committing to that amount of time each day. However, if you really want to boost your practice and flexibility, I would suggest spending as many days as you'd like on each pose until you feel like you've "got it." For some people this might be a few days, for others it may just be 10 minutes.

Another suggestion I'd like for you to keep in mind as you move through each day on your journey, is that if you really want to cut down on your learning curve and the time it takes you to go from newbie to advanced is to practice each yoga pose that you've learned up until this point.

For instance, if you're on Day 4, start your practice with the poses from Day 1, Day 2, Day 3 and so on. This will keep the poses fresh in your mind and also work more parts of your body. Once you get to Day 30 you'll have an entire workout at your disposal.

Again, thank you for purchasing my book and I hope that it helps you to have a better understanding of what yoga is and how it fits into your life. And who knows, maybe you'll love it just as much as I do!

Chapter 1: Yoga 101

Where Did Yoga Come From?

If you're like most people just starting out on their yoga journey then I'm sure you have lots of questions. And we'll get to those, I promise. First, though, I'd like to give you a very brief history of the origins of yoga and summarize how it came to be the yoga we all know and love today.

Yoga is actually a philosophy that came into practice in India about 5,000 years ago! Although it is sometimes part of practicing Buddhism and Hinduism, yoga in and of itself is not a religion.

The founding father of ashtanga yoga and author of the *Yoga Sutras* was Patanjali. Unfortunately, very little is known about who he was or where he came from—or even when exactly he lived. One thing is certain, though—if Patanjali had not completed his *Yoga Sutras* we probably wouldn't know much, if anything, about the yoga we practice today. Patanjali's *Sutras* was a collection of 195 different philosophies about the practice of yoga. His book also outlined the eight individual "limbs" or types of yoga—asana (postures) being the most popular in Western culture.

In the late 19th and early 20th centuries many of the yoga gurus from India introduced yoga as a practice to Western civilization. However, it wasn't until around the 1980's that yoga became a more popular form of physical exercise in the Western world.

Many "serious" yoga practitioners and gurus frown upon our commercialized version of yoga in the United States. The reason for this is because they believe that yoga is meant to be much more than just exercise. Its traditional roots are founded in meditative and spiritual upbringing—becoming in tune to oneself in the process.

I agree with these gurus and in my personal practice I use yoga for spiritual and meditative purposes. However, everyone has to start somewhere. And if you just want to have fun, increase your flexibility and learn some poses along the way I think that's wonderful!

I don't think that yoga needs to be a strict set of standards that only a few people here and there are worthy of experiencing. I think that no matter where you start from, as long as you do, you're going to be better off.

Main Types of Yoga

Aerial—Basically this is yoga...in a hammock! Aerial yoga was introduced in New York and is one of the newest forms of yoga. If you're the adventurous type and already have the more run-of-the-mill yoga classes under your belt then it might be time for you to give this a try.

Ashtanga—This is one of the oldest forms of yoga (remember Patanjali's *Sutras*?) and what we'll be using throughout this book. Ashtanga is made up of six different series' of postures and is used prevalently throughout the West.

Bikram—Bikram yoga was introduced and made popular in the 1970's. Most people looking to lose weight and torch calories during a yoga session turn to Bikram yoga. It's also known as "hot" yoga—and for good reason. The classes are 90 minutes long and consist of a series of 26 poses that are repeated twice during the session. The catch? The room is heated to 104F and a humidity of 40%!

Hatha—Hatha yoga is what all other types of yoga are founded on and uses a more holistic approach than newer variations of yoga. It is a combination of meditation, purification, breathing and postures. It is very gentle and is great for beginners.

Kundalini—This can be one of the most fun forms of yoga, in my opinion. Kundalini yoga is founded on the belief that there is latent energy coiled at the base of our spines and it needs to be released. Kundalini yoga uses meditation and breathing to activate your chakras and release built up energy.

Restorative—This one is pretty self-explanatory. This type of yoga is focused on using different props to restore your physical body with your mental state. It's a very gentle and relaxing form of yoga. It is especially beneficial to those who need to learn to slow down and relieve stress.

Vinyasa—The term Vinyasa originates from the Sanskrit language and actually means "breath-synchronized movement." Which is exactly what you're doing during this type of yoga. You move through a series of poses while at the same time using your exhaling and inhaling breaths to "dance" your way through each pose. It is also sometimes referred to as Vinyasa Flow.

Feel free to experiment and play around with the different types of yoga and find the one that feels best to you. Just because something is deemed "intermediate" or "advanced" doesn't mean you can't try it out. You don't have to limit yourself to beginner types of yoga.

The best thing you can do to figure out where you "belong" in the yoga world is to find a gym or yoga studio that offers bundles—that way you can sample different classes to find the one that fits you best.

Chapter 2: "But I'm Not Flexible"

As a yoga instructor, this is one of the biggest hesitations and objections I hear when it comes to trying yoga—"I'm not flexible."

Well, I'm here to tell you that that is perfectly okay! In fact, it's a wonderful reason to *start* practicing yoga. Do you think that when I first started out I was a super-bendy obscenely flexible human being? I definitely wasn't. I was actually the opposite and it took me almost a year to feel "flexible." Either way, don't be discouraged. Everyone is different and just go at your own pace.

Unfortunately, the older we are and the more we have neglected our physical selves from lack of stretching the longer it takes to get back to being flexible. It doesn't matter if you're an athlete or a couch potato—if you don't incorporate some type of stretching, either through yoga or other body opening exercises you're inevitably going to lose the flexibility we're all born with and even become injured much easier.

It's not enough, though, to just stretch or do yoga every once in awhile. To reap the benefits of flexibility you actually have to stay on top of it and make it an almost-daily habit.

Once you've done it often enough and you increase your flexibility, yoga will become more fun to you. It won't seem like quite as much "work" and you won't have as much of the discomfort as you do in the beginning. Who knows, you may even start to love it and crave doing it every single day like I do!

Modifications

If you have any sort of physical limitations or restrictions I get that yoga can be somewhat intimidating. But it shouldn't be!

Yoga is actually one of the most adaptable and modifiable forms of exercise that exists. For this reason, it's perfect for people who have certain injuries or restrictions. There are even special kinds of yoga just for pregnant women!

Obviously if your physical restriction is a wrist injury then you should avoid putting direct pressure on it. Poses that would cause aggravation to your wrists might include Downward Facing Dog, Four Limbed Staff or Plank Pose. In this situation I would suggest doing a modified version of these poses. How? Simply place your forearms flat on the floor instead of your hands. This will remove the pressure from your wrists and make the moves considerably easier, but still challenging.

You can do this with any sort of restriction and with any pose. If you can't figure out a suitable alternative for you to do the pose comfortably, then just skip it. There is no reason to hurt yourself or cause yourself physical discomfort. In fact, yoga should NEVER be painful. It is a time for relaxation and stress relief and to heal our bodies—not to hurt them.

With any pose in this book you should never go past the point of slight tension. You should feel a good stretch, but it shouldn't hurt. Ever!

Other Common Hang-Ups & Objections

"I Don't Know What I'm Doing"

I truly feel that the best way to learn yoga is by attending a class—especially one geared towards beginners if it's your first time.

The reason for this is because you're sure to learn the poses properly to avoid injury and you can also gain a better understanding of the technique. Not to mention, nothing can beat the feeling you get when you're part of a massive amount of energy like you are when taking a yoga class.

However, I get that not everyone is at a place in their hearts and minds to feel comfortable practicing yoga in front of others. That's why I created this book! You don't have to know what you're doing, you just have to follow along and commit to some positive change.

"I Don't Have Anything to Wear"

Yes, we all want to look our best. However, that's the beauty of practicing yoga at home—you don't have to dress for a fashion show and you don't have to worry about who's going to see you.

If you do attend a class and you're stressed about what to wear there are a few things to keep in mind:

- Wear clothes that fit you properly (avoid loose tops where everything is hanging out or too-small clothing items that you'll constantly be pulling at)
- Pick an outfit that allows you to move freely
- No need to bring shoes or even socks

Aside from these few guidelines there really isn't any need to worry about your clothing choice—I assure you most people aren't paying attention.

"I Don't Live Near a Yoga Studio"

You don't need to! You can start exactly where you are: at home, with this book. And once you finish this book I'll have plenty of others waiting.

There are also great resources online for free yoga tutorial videos and classes you can do at home. YouTube is a wonderful site to access free yoga classes. One of my favorite channels is Yoga By Candace—she has a wide variety of videos for all experience levels and they're free.

If you're looking for a website that offers yoga videos DoYogaWithMe.com is 100% free and has plenty of content to keep you occupied.

"I'm Not Religious, or Even Spiritual For That Matter"

That's completely fine. No one is going to try and change you or "convert" you. Yoga is not a religion. It's true that a lot of the yoga practices are founded in spiritual philosophies and traditions, but that shouldn't deter you from attending a class or practicing at home.

Spirituality looks different for each and every person. At the deepest level, yoga is about simply connecting with yourself and finding inner peace and awareness. You don't have to label yourself as religious or spiritual to gain these benefits and no one expects you to.

"Yoga is For Girls"

Really, guys? It's 2015. This is the best that you can come up with? I feel like I shouldn't even address this hang-up because it's completely ridiculous, but I'll simply say this: **men** were the first to practice yoga. Remember Patanjali?

Are most modern classes in the Western world full of women? Yes. Should that stop you? No. If you're truly that concerned about it being "for girls" then try BrogaYoga. Or as mentioned previously you can practice yoga at home if it makes you uncomfortable to be surrounded by women.

In case you haven't caught on: there's never a good excuse **not** to practice yoga!

Chapter 3: Common Yoga Lingo

I know that for a lot of people, yoga can be intimidating just because there are so many new and overwhelmingly long words and terminologies for everything. Not to mention a lot of it is in Sanskrit (an ancient Indic language originating in India). When you throw a foreign language in there it makes it that much scarier.

Not only do you have to learn all these new poses, but you have to learn all these foreign phrases, too. Well—I promise it's not that complicated. And you don't even need to know the specific yoga terms to reap the benefits of practicing yoga. In time, though, the knowledge will come to you.

Until then, I've compiled a basic dictionary of the most prevalent terms and what they mean. Please keep in mind that these are very simplistic definitions. If you're interested in learning more about a term or idea please research it further to get a more complete understanding of the subject.

Sanskrit Yoga Dictionary

Ahimsa—Non-violence/non-injury (yama).

Ananda—A slow and gentle type of yoga that uses affirmations along with the asanas.

Anusara—A type of yoga that is heart-oriented and combines alignment of your body with energy-filled asanas.

Aparigraha—Non-selfishness (yama).

Asanas—Most commonly it refers to yoga postures.

Ashram—A secluded place where yoga and meditation are taught.

Ashtanga—One of the most common forms of yoga, it is physically challenging and helps with flexibility, strength and stamina.

Asmita—Represents your ego and individuality.

Asteya—Non-stealing (yama).

Bikram—A strenuous type of yoga in a very high temperature room.

Brahmacharya—Purity, non-lust (yama).

Brahman—Representation of God.

Buddhi—The intellect.

Chakras—The 7 sources of life force and energy that radiate from the spinal column from the crown of the head to the base of your spine.

Dharana—Literally means "to hold firm," mindfulness.

Dharma—Self-discipline and doing the right thing.

Dhyana—The process of meditating to quiet the mind.

Guru—Spiritual teacher.

Hatha—The yoga style of physical well-being that focuses on centering the mind, body and spirit.

Ishvar-pranidhana—Center of the Divine (niyama).

Karma—Destiny or fate based on a person's actions.

Kundalini—Cosmic energy inside our body that is coiled at the base of the spine, waiting to be awakened.

Kundalini yoga—The focus is your breathing and chanting to awaken and release your Kundalini energy.

Mandala—A geometric circle that represents one's spiritual journey, often referred to as a labyrinth.

Mantra—A sacred chant.

Meditation—Practice of guiding your focus inward to achieve inner peace.

Mudras—Different hand gestures believed to direct life current throughout the body.

Namaste—Translated from Sanskrit it means, "The divine light within me salutes the divine light within you." It's a friendly greeting that is supposed to represent our soul connecting to another soul through our heart chakra.

Niyamas—Outlined in Patanjali's *Yoga Sutras* as the 5 observances of inner discipline.

Om/Aum—Vibration of the Universe, often chanted during meditation or yoga.

Prana—Life force or energy—also referred to as 'chi' in Chinese culture.

Pranayama—The practice of breath control.

Pratyahara—The practice of dulling the senses to still the mind during meditation.

Santosha—Contentment (niyama).

Satya—Honesty and truthfulness (yama).

Samadhi—State of super-consciousness, pure bliss.

Shanti—This means 'peace.' In Buddhism and Hinduism you chant 'shanti' three consecutive times in order to promote peace in body, mind and speech.

Shauca—Purity inside and out (niyama).

Shodhana—Cleansing ritual.

Svadhyaya—Self-reflection about your own nature and beliefs and how it fits into the Universe's spiritual journey (niyama).

Swami—Respectful title for a guru.

Tantra—Type of yoga that practices strong breath techniques combined with visualization, chanting and asana to release Kundalini energy.

Tapas—Self-discipline (niyama).

Ujjayi—A type of breathing exercise that, when you inhale, creates sound in your throat.

Vinyasa—A type of yoga that is a continuous flow of movement where postures are linked with breath work.

Yamas—Defined in Patanjali's *Yoga Sutras* as 5 yamas (moral conduct): non-stealing, non-possessiveness, moderation, honesty/truth and non-violence.

Yoga—Yoga literally means yoke or union. This is why yoga represents the practice of connecting our body, mind and spirit as one—not just with ourselves but with the Universe as well. It all becomes inter-connected.

Yogi/Yogini—A person who practices yoga. Yogini is the female form.

Please note: you do not have to be a walking dictionary for all of these terms in order to practice and be good at yoga. This is just included for your reference because I personally think that the history and roots of yoga are very important. Knowing more about what I'm practicing has given me a higher level of understanding and satisfaction from my practice of yoga.

I promise if you spend the time learning and growing in the culture of yoga you will be rewarded ten-fold through much greater levels of self-awareness and spirituality.

Chapter 4: Benefits of Yoga

The benefits of yoga are pretty much limitless. I mean, where do I even begin? It's hard to narrow it down because there are so many benefits that can't be described. I mean, yes, of course there are all of the health benefits that most people know about, but so many of the best things about yoga are hard to put into words—it's an internal shift of your human vibration. Yoga has helped me look beyond myself, to change my focus so that it's more about the needs of others and the greater good of the Universe and human race.

All of this sounds cheesy, I'm sure, but if you stick with practicing yoga long enough I'm sure you'll begin to understand what I mean.

If you're more interested in the benefits that *can* be put into words then keep reading, I've got you covered.

Improves Lung Capacity & Breathing

If you're a yogi, then overall you're going to take deeper breaths—this is much more efficient and calming than the traditional shallow breathing technique that most people develop. By utilizing this type of breathing you are increasing the oxygen levels in your blood significantly.

Also, the breathing techniques in yoga promote breathing through your nose, which is actually healthier since you're filtering the air of all its dirt and dander that would otherwise go into your lungs.

Promotes Deeper Sleep

Too much stimulation is definitely a bad thing and yoga gives you relief from the stress and fast pace of every day life. One of the best types of yoga to practice for a better night's sleep is Restorative yoga.

Releases Tension

We all have bad habits that actually lead to muscle fatigue, soreness and chronic tension—all of which can put you in a bad mood. The longer you practice yoga the easier it will be for you to identify where exactly in your body you tend to hold tension and it will also slowly help you to rid yourself of these habits.

Improves Balance& Posture

By regularly practicing yoga it helps you to become more aware of where your body is at in relation to space at any given moment. Because of this it means you'll automatically achieve a better sense of balance. Did you know that when you have better balance you're also going to have better posture? Yes, it's true. And if you're anything like me then you definitely need help in this area. Most of us spend the majority of our days sitting and slouching—yoga can help with that!

Promotes Relaxation

Because yoga promotes relaxation and slow breathing techniques, it actually helps you carry these habits over into your everyday life. The reason this is a good thing is that it shifts your nervous system and utilizes the parasympathetic nervous system instead of the sympathetic. If you're unsure why that's a good thing, suffice it to say that it simply makes you more calm.

Keeps You Focused

Yoga, as you know, helps you to focus on the present moment. If you practice yoga regularly then the benefits are going to compound and you'll have a better memory, improved coordination and reaction times and even a higher IQ! Why? Because through yoga you have learned to be less distracted by your thoughts.

Increases Muscle Strength

If you believe yoga is a lazy person's exercise, then I'm sorry but you'd be way wrong! Yoga can be an incredibly challenging and toning form of exercise all combined with the added benefit of flexibility. Sure you can build up your muscles in the gym all day, but when it comes down to it you're not going to be much more flexible.

Keeps Your Spine Healthy

Did you know that the spinal disks can only get the nutrients they need with movement? That's right. So if you're sitting all day with little to no movement it's a recipe for disaster for your spine. But there's an easy fix: yoga! If you're doing a well-rounded yoga routine with lots of forward bends, twists and even backbends you're sure to keep the nutrients flowing and your spinal disks well oiled.

Promotes Lymph Health & Immunity

Because yoga combines lots of stretching and movement with its different poses and postures you're sure to be moving your organs and muscles regularly. This is good because it keeps your lymph system flowing which helps to obliterate cancer cells, get rid of toxic waste and fight infection. Impressive!

Increases Happiness

You might not know it, but yoga can actually relieve depression. That's right! If you practice yoga regularly you can increase your serotonin levels and decrease cortisol—all of which means a happier you.

Improves Self-Esteem

Before I started practicing yoga I didn't feel very good about myself. I was always pointing out my own flaws and constantly bombarding myself with hateful comments day after day. Because of this I had incredibly low self-esteem and in turn it only made me treat myself worse—by eating foods I knew were bad for me, not getting enough sleep...you get the picture.

And as cliché as it may sound, yoga changed all that. Obviously it didn't happen overnight, but as I found myself returning to yoga I realized it was because it made me feel better about myself—good even and I think that we all could stand to benefit from more positive feelings like that.

Decreases Pain

This is one of my favorite benefits of practicing yoga! Quite a few years ago I was hit by a car while crossing at a crosswalk—although I was lucky enough not to break any bones (thank you, Universe!) my lower back was in an enormous amount of pain.

Yoga has completely turned all of that around for me and for many many others as well. It's not just back pain, though: people with fibromyalgia, arthritis, carpal tunnel and other chronic pain conditions have all seen improvement through regular practice of yoga.

Provides You With Inner Strength

Through practicing yoga it gives you a sense of discipline that you didn't know you had before. It helps you overcome other bad habits in your life without even making a conscious effort or decision to change them. Without even thinking about it, as a direct result of practicing yoga, you may slowly start to eliminate habits that are innately bad for you even if you had a hard time doing so in the past.

Relationships Improve

Yoga actually helps to cultivate health and healing through your relationships. Why? Because the longer you practice yoga you learn to develop certain traits that make you better (e.g. compassion, friendliness, selflessness). Not only that, but in turn your sex life will become better as well. You'll be more confident and outgoing—and not to mention more flexible!

So what does this all boil down to? If you expect change and expect to become better, then you will be. You just have to be open to receiving the benefits that yoga has to offer. If you open your heart and mind to all that it provides, I promise you won't be disappointed.

Chapter 5: Tips for Beginners

In this chapter we're going to go over some tips and hints that I wish I would have known when I first started practicing yoga over 13 years ago. When I began my yoga journey I really didn't have a mentor or anyone to turn to for advice. And back in 2002 it wasn't nearly as popular or prevalent as it is now—hooray for change!

So without further ado, here is my advice to you, new Yogi...

Enjoy Being a Beginner

So many times in life we are focused on becoming "the best." We strive for perfection in everything and all of this is at the expense of our enjoyment. I wish I had learned to slow down just a little bit and relish in the fact that I was a novice! I promise no one is analyzing your every move or judging you for being a beginner. It just doesn't happen. So relax and be still in the moment.

And this might seem obvious, but...you're not going to be a beginner forever. Embrace all the silliness and newness of everything and just soak up all the knowledge with a smile on your face. Also, don't be afraid to ask questions—if you don't know what 'pranayama' is or you forget how to do a certain pose—ask! Or if you're practicing at home, research. The Internet is an amazing tool that we have access to. There's no reason for you to go without getting the answers you're looking for.

Avoid Comparison

It's true what Theodore Roosevelt said: "Comparison is the thief of joy." This can be especially true as a newbie taking a class for the first time, but heck, even advanced yogis can fall prey to comparing themselves to others. It's easy to do in any aspect of your life.

But here's the good news: if you're focusing on your practice and your inner mindset you don't have time to compare. And not only that but the more you practice yoga the better you'll get at loving yourself and being okay where you're at. It's all about the present. The truth is, there will be certain people every now and then in all areas of your life that are going to judge you and maybe even make you feel uncomfortable. And guess what? You can't change them, but you can change yourself and how it makes you feel.

So if you do happen to be in a class with someone who appears judgmental or disapproving, brush it off. Hold your head high and focus on bettering *you*—after all, that's what you're practicing yoga for anyway.

As a side note, I realize that we live in the snap-happy 21st century where Instagram prevails and it seems like everyone is posting pictures of himself or herself in a crazy new yoga pose every single day. It's easy to want to compare yourself to your favorite Instagram yogi—especially when it seems like it all just comes so naturally and effortlessly to them. Try to remember, though, that what you're seeing is a tiny moment of where they are in their practice. It has probably taken them years to get to this point and who knows how many pictures they had to take before they got the pose just right? So try not to be too hard on yourself.

Respect Your Body

Oftentimes, especially when just starting out, it's natural for us to have preconceived notions about how deep we should be able to get into a pose or what we should look like when we do them. But please please remember: yoga is **not** about what you look like when you're in a pose; it's about **how you feel.**

Don't let your ego get in the way of the experience and the feeling of being present with your body. Don't force your body to move in ways that it isn't yet comfortable with—you should never be in pain when practicing yoga.

If you are, you're pushing yourself too hard and you need to back off a little. Listen to your inner voice and the limits of your physical self, push slightly past where you feel comfortable. This is how you will grow in your practice, but you won't run the risk of injuring yourself.

Also, there's no set rule as to how often you should practice yoga. Just listen to and respect your body. It will let you know when it needs a break and when it's ready for more.

Focus on Your Breath

This is one of the most important facets of yoga, hands down. You'll be able to tell when you've pushed yourself too far if your breathing becomes labored or jagged and uneven.

Back off until you can once again resume the steady flow of breath. The breath is the life force of yoga and if you're restricting it then you're not doing yoga.

Let the Om's Flow

I remember when I first started practicing yoga I was so scared to chant and do the mantras. I'm a naturally quiet person so it was rather intimidating for me. I see the same thing in my classes that I teach. Almost always there's hesitation there— almost as if it's wrong or they're going to get in trouble.

32

Don't be scared! Let it all out. You're vibrating in tune with the Universe and you are not alone. This simple, albeit uncomfortable at first, practice is an amazing reflection of the greater vibration of the Universe and how everything connects as one. It's an incredibly powerful experience—especially if you let go and just be.

Have FUN

It's very easy to get caught up in all of the technicalities of yoga, but you should strive for a carefree simplicity.

There's no need to stress over all of the pronunciations or whether you should do this pose or that pose. Do what feels good! Do what feels natural. It all comes down to how you feel and you should always be having fun.

If you need an icebreaker on how to let loose and get your flow going try a Kundalini class. After that you should never feel out of place or uncomfortable again.

Get a Yoga Mat—and Possibly Other Equipment

Now, I don't want any of what I'm about to say deter you from starting your yoga practice. You can and certainly should start right where you're at, right now, with what you've already got.

However, if you're going to practice yoga long-term and make it a hobby then I do suggest purchasing a few helpful tools of the trade.

First and foremost you need a yoga mat. They sell these virtually everywhere now and you should be able to find one quite easily. However, my suggestion would be to invest in one with quite a bit of foam. I see lots of thin yoga mats that look like nothing more than a shelf liner and it's not conducive for a lot of the poses.

They don't provide enough padding and it often prevents the proper form of certain poses—especially on wood floors.

My second recommendation would be to get a couple yoga blocks. These are especially beneficial to less flexible people and beginners. They alleviate tension and provide comfort in some of the more complex poses that aren't so easy when you're first starting out.

There's plenty of other gadgets out there, but I think that just starting out you don't need to overcomplicate things—stick to the basics and you'll be fine.

Be Open to Advice

Sometimes it's hard to take advice, especially if we feel like we're being criticized or judged. If you're taking a class and the instructor offers guidance to you, try not to take it personally.

Speaking from experience, instructors are only looking out for their students and we want them to get the most out of our class. We don't correct your posture or point out a mistake to embarrass you—we do it because we truly care.

If you find it happens a lot and it really bothers you try giving your instructor a heads-up after class. Simply let them know that it messes up your flow and you'd appreciate it if they would refrain from calling you out in class.

Most instructors will be more than understanding.

Don't Give Up

Plenty of times I've seen someone come in to a beginner's yoga class and feel like they just don't "get" it. They feel like there's something wrong with them if their pose doesn't look exactly like mine or they can't go quite as deep.

I understand that it can be frustrating, but try not to have expectations of how you should be or look. Especially in the beginning. Focus on your breathing and how you're feeling. Yoga should not stress you out and if it does, something's not right. Either you need to adjust your state of mind or erase your expectations or maybe you need to ease off your intensity level.

But no matter what, don't quit after your first experience with yoga—whether it's at home or in a studio, keep going. There are going to be some rough patches and bumps along the way, as with anything. It's going to take hard work and practice to get better, but try and remember to enjoy the journey and the process and not be so hard on yourself.

It Doesn't Always Need to Be "Go Hard or Go Home" (Restorative vs. Vinyasa)

There are plenty of people (yogis and non-yogis, alike) who believe that Restorative yoga is not as beneficial or healthy as Vinyasa Flow yoga.

Don't get me wrong—Vinyasa Flow is intense physically, but Restorative is as equally as intense mentally. So just because you're not sweating and grunting and feeling the burn it doesn't mean that you're not working hard.

One of the things I love about yoga is the fact that it is a mental challenge and provides an escape from the rigors of everyday life. Whether it's in the form of physical sweat, or mental sweat they're both beneficial and have their place in yoga.

You Might Get a Little Emotional

Whether you're aware of it or not, we store a lot of emotional energy in our physical bodies, especially in the hip and shoulder areas.

When you practice yoga you open up these areas and release a lot of the pent up emotions and energy that reside there. This is why it's sometimes unsettling to perform certain poses that open your hips and shoulders—but this isn't a bad thing. It's actually quite the opposite. It gives our bodies a chance to release from whatever we've been holding onto.

However, sometimes this can mean after an especially intense and opening yoga session you may have unexplainable outbursts of emotions and maybe even tears. Let it flow through you and pass out the other side. Feel the emotion and then let it go so you can make room for positivity and love.

Never Skip Savasana

This is actually my number one pet peeve: students who leave class without completing Savasana (Corpse Pose). Yes, it's an easy pose and you're ready to go about the rest of your day, I get it. But it's so much more than that!

When you skip out on Savasana at the end of your yoga session you are bypassing the most important thing: the processing of all that you've just been through. If you don't give your body and nervous system time to come back together as one and reflect on the last 60 minutes or so and all that you've learned then you're not going to get the complete benefit out of the session you've just had.

It's just a few minutes and I'm sure that you'll notice the difference it makes in the clarity of your mindset when you're done.

Chapter 6: The Poses

Now for the part we've all been waiting for: the asanas (poses)! As I mentioned earlier on in the book, please remember that you should go at your own pace. If you feel like 10 minutes is enough for you each day that's wonderful and you'll get a solid base level introduction to practicing yoga. However, if you prefer to spend more time on each pose I highly recommend it.

As you get more comfortable do each pose that you've learned up until the day you are on. For instance, if you're on Day 5: do all poses 1-4 up until Day 5 so that they stay fresh in your memory and you can build on the flexibility you're developing with each pose.

Ready? Let's get started.

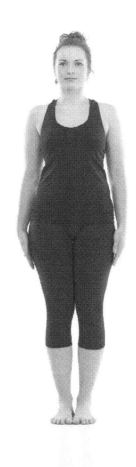

Day 1: Mountain Pose

This pose might look like you're just standing there, but if done correctly it serves a much greater purpose and is generally the starting position for other standing poses.

Step 1: Stand upright so that your big toes are completely flat and touching the floor. Keep your feet about hip width apart and parallel to one another. Now, flex your toes upward and wide—really stretch. This is going to gauge whether or not you're balancing your posture correctly. If you lose balance then most likely you're not centering your weight evenly on all points of your feet so you need to correct your balance so that it's spread evenly on your feet.

Step 2: Contract your thigh muscles and try to lift your kneecaps, but do so without contracting your lower abdomen. Lift the inside of your ankles to help strengthen those inner arches and visualize an imaginary line of energy that spreads the length of your inner thighs to your groin and then from your core (or torso) to your neck, head—all the way out exiting through the crown of your head. Now turn your upper thighs slightly inward and visualize lengthening the tailbone down to the floor while lifting your pubic bone toward your belly button.

Step 3: Now focus on pressing your shoulder blades back and then slowly stretch them out and release down your back. Lift the upper part of your sternum toward the ceiling without pushing the lower part of your ribs outward. Widen and stretch the collarbones, then hang your arms at your sides, palms facing forward.

Step 4: Finally, balance your head completely above the center of your pelvic area. Make sure that your chin is parallel to the floor and keep your mouth and throat soft as well as your eyes.

Stay here and breathe slowly and intentionally for 1 minute or however long you feel comfortable.

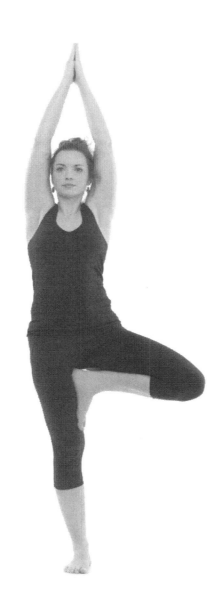

Day 2: Tree Pose

Step 1: First, stand in Mountain pose and begin to shift your weight a little bit onto your left foot. Keep the inside of the foot firm on the floor and bend the right knee. Slowly reach down and grab your right ankle with your right hand.

Step 2: Pull your right foot up and place it against your inner left thigh as high as you can to where it feels comfortable. Your goal should eventually be to press your right heel into your left groin completely flat with your toes pressing down toward the floor. Keep your pelvic bone directly over your left foot.

Step 3: Visualize lengthening your tailbone, getting it as long as you can. Press your right foot into your inner thigh and then place your hands in the prayer position in front of you, looking straight ahead.

If you don't want to put your hands in prayer position you can place them on your hips or at your sides.

Stay in this position for 1 minute, breathing evenly. After you've completed this, go back to Mountain pose and do Tree pose with your opposite leg.

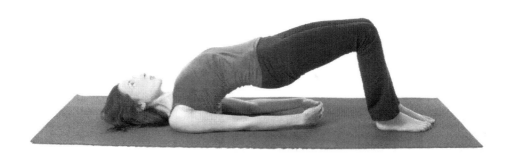

Day 3: Bridge Pose

Step 1: Begin by lying flat on your back. Bring your knees up to a 90-degree angle and place your feet flat on the floor with your heels as close to your glutes as possible.

Step 2: Exhale while pressing your feet and arms firmly into the floor, contract your tailbone up toward your pubic bone and firm your buttocks muscles. Now lift your butt off the floor keeping everything parallel.

Step 3: Place your hands below your back on the floor either flat or you can clasp them together if that's more comfortable. Keep your abdomen muscles engaged and try to lengthen your back.

Step 4: Keep your chin lifted slightly above your sternum and your shoulder blades firm. To keep your shoulders from closing in, firm your outer arms and broaden the shoulder blades, stretching them across the base of your neck.

Stay in this pose for 1 minute and when you're ready to come out of it, do so by exhaling and rolling each of your vertebrae slowly down onto the floor.

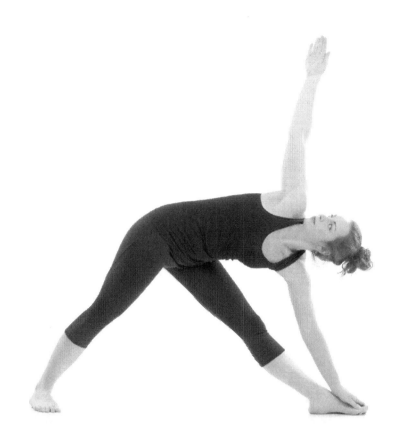

Day 4: Extended Triangle Pose

Step 1: Stand in Mountain pose and as you exhale, spread your legs about 3-4 feet apart. Place your arms in the air parallel to the floor and then reach out to your sides, shoulders wide, and palms facing down.

Step 2: Position your left foot slightly to the right and then place your right foot at 90 degrees. Rotate your right thigh so that it's facing outward and the center of your right knee is in line with your ankle.

Step 3: Now, exhale and bend your torso to the right placing it over your right leg. Do not bend at the waist, but rather at your hip. Strengthen your left leg and press your left heel into the floor. Rotate your torso to the left and let your left hip move forward a bit.

Step 4: Next you can rest your right hand however is comfortable—on the floor, your ankle, shin, etc. Now, stretch and raise your left arm up high to the ceiling lining it up with your shoulders. Be sure to keep your head neutral or you can turn to the left to look up at your left thumb.

Stay in this pose for 1 minute and then slowly inhale and come out of it by raising your arm toward the ceiling and pressing your back heel into the floor. Follow the same steps for your opposite side.

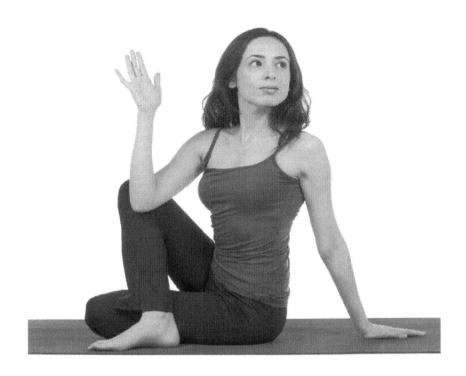

Day 5: Half Twist

Step 1: Sit on the floor with your legs flat in front of you. Bend your left knee and place your left leg over your right so that your left foot is resting on the floor at the edge of your right hip.

Step 2: Now, move your right foot over your left knee so that it's positioned outside of the thigh. Be sure to keep both sides of your butt evenly on the ground.

Step 3: Next you're going to lean back onto your right hand and then inhale while place your left arm over your head to lengthen your torso and spine.

Step 4: As you exhale twist to your right and bring your left elbow outside of the right thigh. Look over your right shoulder and be sure to keep length in your neck. As you continue to inhale try to lengthen your spine more. As you exhale, twist deeper into the pose.

Stay in this position, inhaling and exhaling for 1 minute. As you come out of the pose, do it on the exhale and release gently. Switch to the opposite side.

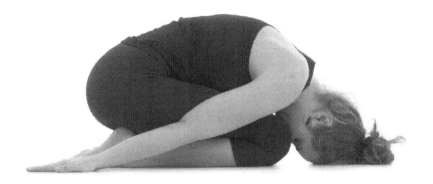

Day 6: Child's Pose

Step 1: Get into a kneeling position on the floor and sit back on your heels. Separate your knees hip width apart.

Step 2: As you exhale, lay your torso down on the mat between your thighs. Once you're settled in, lengthen the tailbone and neck.

Step 3: Now you can position your hands either straight out in front of you, palms toward the ground or you can place them at your sides palms facing up. Whatever is most comfortable to you. After all, this is a resting pose.

Relax in this position for 1 minute or longer, releasing the tension in all areas of your body.

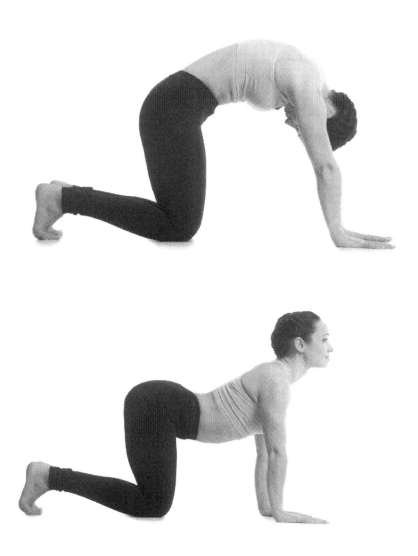

Day 7: Cat-Cow

Step 1: Start with both hands and knees on the floor. Be sure to keep your knees under the hips and wrists under the shoulders. Your spine should be neutral and back flat. Keep your abdominal muscles engaged and breath in deeply.

Step 2: As you exhale, round the spine upward as far as you can towards the ceiling. It helps if you imagine pulling your belly button into your spine. At the same time pull your chin into your chest and relax your neck. This would be considered the cat pose.

Step 3: When you inhale, arch the back and relax your stomach, keeping everything loose. Raise your head and tailbone upward making sure not to add pressure to your neck. This would be considered the cow pose.

Step 4: Flow back and forth from cat to cow for as long as you like, just be sure to connect the movements with your breathing and really stay conscious of each vertebrae as you inhale and exhale.

Again, you can do this for as long as you wish. It's a great spinal warming exercise and helps alleviate low back pain. I recommend at least 1 minute.

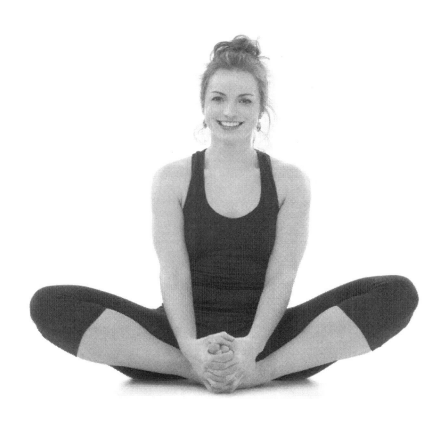

Day 8: Bound Angle Pose

Step 1: Begin by sitting on the floor with your legs out in front of you. Exhale as you bend the knees and bring your heels inward to your pelvis. Lower your knees out to the sides and press your feet together.

Step 2: The idea is to bring your heels inward as much as you can without it hurting. Once you've found your spot grab your big toes with your fingers.

Step 3: You should be sitting upright with your pelvic bone in a neutral position. Keep your shoulders back and your torso up as you lengthen your body.

Step 4: Don't try to force your knees toward the floor, but rather focus on pushing your thighbones into the floor.
Stay here for at least 1 minute, preferably closer to 3 minutes.

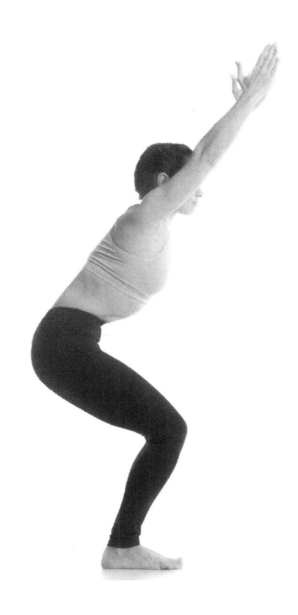

Day 9: Chair Pose

Step 1: Begin in Mountain pose. As you inhale, bring your arms perpendicular to the ground. You can clasp your hands together or you can keep your arms parallel, palms inward—whatever is most comfortable.

Step 2: As you exhale, bend the knees and bring your thighs as parallel to the ground as possible. Your knees will be over your feet and torso will be slightly forward above the thighs until you're at a right angle with the tops of your thighs. Press your thighbones down into your heels.

Step 3: Keep your shoulder blades firm and push your tailbone down toward the ground and inward to your pubic bone. Try to keep your lower back elongated.

Stay in this position for 1 minute. Inhale and lift your arms, as you exhale release and bring your body back into Mountain pose.

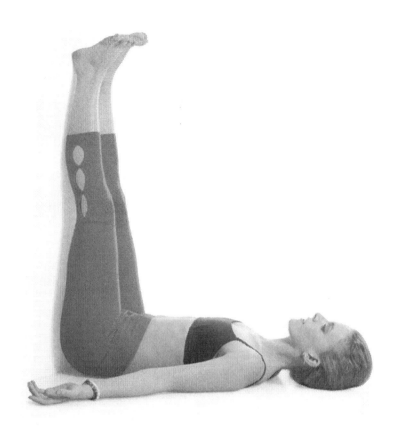

Day 10: Legs-Up-The-Wall Pose

Step 1: Determine the distance you need to be from the wall: if you're tall move farther away, if you're shorter get closer and adjust as needed. If you feel like this pose puts too much pressure on your lower back or you're uncomfortable, you can use a rolled up towel or a bolster to provide support in your lower back.

Step 2: Sit sideways and start with your right side facing the wall, as you exhale, swiftly bring your legs up onto the wall in one fluid movement and then slowly lower your shoulders and head onto the floor. If you feel like you need support at the base of your neck feel free to place a rolled up towel or wash cloth there to ease the pressure.

Step 3: Be mindful of the position of your chin—make sure you're not pushing it into your chest. Keep your shoulders pressed down flat towards the floor and place your arms out at your sides, palms facing upward.

Step 4: Keep the legs slightly taut to keep them from "drooping" and then sink the weight of your lower body down toward your pelvic floor.

Stay in this pose for as long as you like—it's exceptionally comfortable for getting into a meditative state. Just be sure that when you come out of the pose you're not twisting your back, but rather roll gently to one side instead.

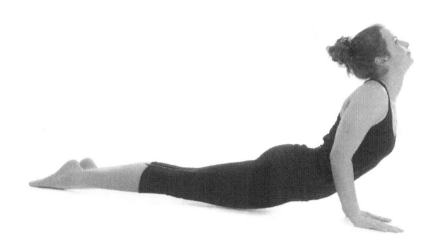

Day 11: Cobra Pose

Step 1: Lie on your stomach in the floor with your legs out behind you and the tops of your feet touching the floor. Next, place your hands on the floor directly under your shoulders as you press your elbows back and into your sides.

Step 2: Place pressure on the tops of your feet and thighs and pubic bone as you press yourself firmly into the floor. As you inhale, straighten your arms and lift your chest off the floor. Make sure that you don't go so far that you're pubic bone is off the floor.

Step 3: Keep your shoulder blades firm as you "puff" your chest forward, lifting through the top of your sternum. Be mindful not to tighten your lower back. If you notice quite a bit of lower back pain or pressure, feel free to widen the distance between your legs as this should help.

Stay in this pose for 30 seconds as you continue to breathe slowly and evenly. On the exhale you can release.

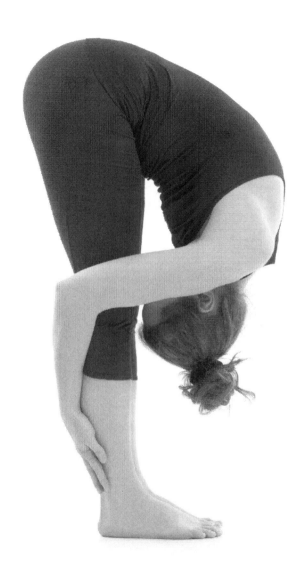

Day 12: Standing Forward Bend

Step 1: Stand in Mountain pose with your hands on your hips. As you exhale, bend slowly forward at your hips. At the same time you should be drawing your stomach inward and engaging your abdominal muscles. You want to focus on lengthening your mid-section as you descend.

Step 2: Now, with your knees as straight as you can keep them, place your fingertips or palms on the floor in front of you. If this is too much of a stretch just grab wherever you can reach to—maybe your ankles or even your calves. Remember not to push yourself too hard.

Step 3: Press your heels into the floor and lift your butt into the air. As you inhale, focus on lengthening your mid-section. As you exhale release yourself deeper into the forward bend.

Step 4: Be mindful of your neck and keep it loose—let it hang freely.

Stay in this pose for 1 minute and then gently bring yourself out of it by unrolling your torso as you inhale.

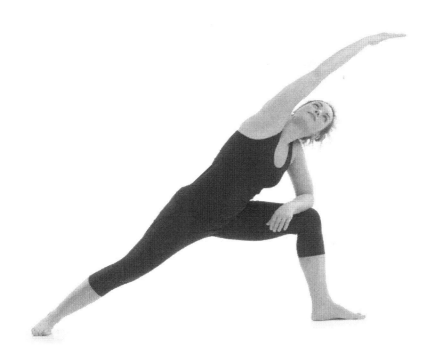

Day 13: Extended Side Angle

This pose is somewhat similar to the Extended Triangle—the difference being that instead of both legs staying straight you will come down into a lunge position with the leg you're leaning into.

Step 1: Stand in Mountain pose and as you exhale, spread your legs about 3-4 feet apart. Place your arms in the air parallel to the floor and then reach out to your sides, shoulders wide, and palms facing down.

Step 2: Rotate your right thigh outward and keep your kneecap in line with your right ankle. Now, you're going to roll your left hip forward and to the right, but make sure you're upper torso goes back and to the left.

Step 3: Firmly keep your left heel planted into the floor and as you exhale bend your right knee into a lunge position over your right ankle, making sure not to go past your toes. Try to aim for your right thigh being parallel to the floor.

Step 4: Keep your shoulder blades firm and extend your left arm up to the ceiling, turning your palm to face your head. As you inhale, reach your left arm over your left ear. Focus on stretching and lengthening your entire left side of your body. As you do so, look up at your left arm and also be mindful to lengthen your right side of your torso as well.

Step 5: As you exhale press the right side of your mid-section down onto your right thigh and press the fingertips of your right hand onto the floor. Your right thigh should be parallel with the floor.

Stay here and breathe for 1 minute, focusing on staying as open as possible. Reverse your feet and do the same thing for your left side.

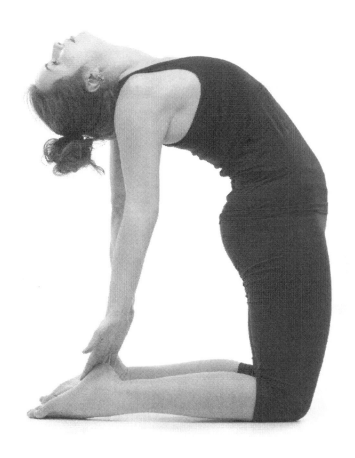

Day 14: Camel Pose

Step 1: Get on the floor with your knees hip width apart. Visualize yourself drawing your glutes up into your body, but keep your hips soft while you plant your shins and tops of the feet into the floor.

Step 2: Place your hands on your hips as you rest your palms on your butt with your fingers pointing down. As you inhale, keep your shoulder blades pressed back and your head high. Ideally you want to keep your thighs perpendicular to the floor, but if you're a beginner it's perfectly okay to give yourself some slack. If you can't go straight back to touch your feet you can turn slightly to one side and place your hand on your foot, then go back to the neutral position and place your other hand on your other foot.

Step 3: Make sure to lift your pelvic bone upward and focus on lengthening your spine and releasing pressure. As you do so place your hands against your heels and your fingers pointing down to your toes. Don't squeeze your shoulder blades together and don't tighten your neck or throat area.

Stay in this pose for up to 1 minute, however long is comfortable to you. If you feel pressure in your lower back you can counteract this pose by going into Child's pose for a minute or so.

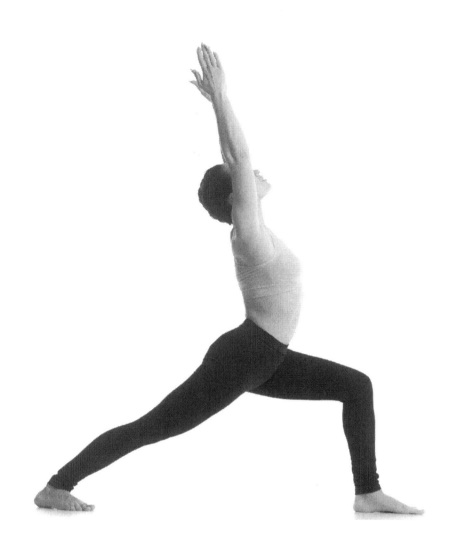

Day 15: Warrior I

Step 1: Start off in Mountain pose and then exhale as you bring your left foot back behind you 3-4 feet. Now, turn your left foot outward to 45 degrees as you keep your right foot forward.

Step 2: Make sure to keep both of your hips facing forward and parallel to the floor as you bring your shoulders forward as well. Inhale and then raise both arms perpendicular to the floor. Be sure to keep them open and shoulder width apart.

Step 3: Reach up towards your fingertips and face your palms inwards while pulling your shoulders back away from your neck. As you exhale engage your ab muscles and bring your pelvic bone down.

Step 4: Carefully move your right knee forward and align the knee over the heel. Keep breathing and make sure the pressure is located in your right heel and not your toes.

Step 5: Be sure to keep your head neutral by either looking forward or by tilting your head back to look up toward your thumbs.

Stay in this pose for up to 1 minute and then repeat on the opposite side.

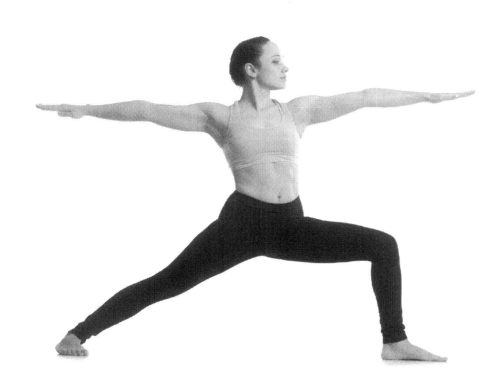

Day 16: Warrior II

Step 1: Start off in Mountain pose and then exhale as you bring your left foot back behind you 3-4 feet. Now, turn your left foot outward to 90 degrees as you move your hips out toward the left and your right knee moves over the center of the right ankle.

Step 2: As you inhale, raise your arms parallel to the floor above your thighs. As you do so keep your shoulder blades wide and open up your chest as you face your palms downward. When you exhale, bend your right knee over your right heel and make sure your balance is evenly dispersed.

Step 3: Tuck your tailbone under and toward the pubic bone. Keep stretching your arms wide and parallel to the ground. Don't lean to your right; keep your sternum tall and neutral.

Step 4: Your eyes should be focused over your right arm to your middle finger.

Stay in this pose for up to 1 minute and then repeat on the opposite side.

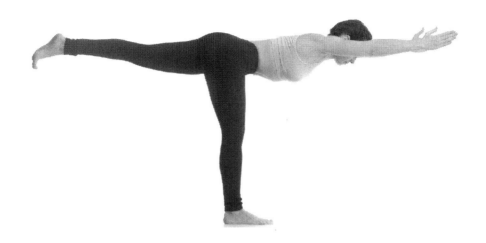

Day 17: Warrior III

Step 1: Start off in Mountain pose and then exhale as you bring your left foot back behind you 2 feet. You should keep your weight focused over your right foot and your toes facing forward.

Step 2: As you move your hands to your hips make sure the hips and shoulders are aligned perpendicular to the floor. Focus on drawing your belly button into your waist, then inhale and bring your left foot off the ground while you lean forward at the hips.

Step 3: Stare straight down as you bend forward from your hips and move yourself parallel to the floor. Be careful not to lock your knees and stop once your hips are aligned.

Step 4: If you want to practice more balance you can stretch your arms out in front of you or to your sides.

Stay in this pose for 5-10 breaths and then repeat for the opposite side.

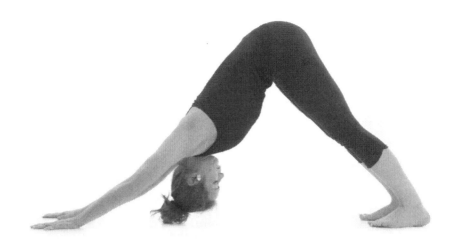

Day 18: Downward Facing Dog

Step 1: Get on the floor on your hands and knees so that your knees are right below the hips and your hands are slightly in front of your shoulders as you keep your toes pointed under.

Step 2: As you exhale, bring your knees away from the mat and keep a slight bend as you lift your heels away from the mat. Focus on lengthening you tailbone and gently press it toward your pubic bone. Lift your butt high toward the ceiling and bring your ankles into the groin.

Step 3: On another exhale stretch your heels down to the mat and straighten your knees—but don't lock them. Keep your arms firm and press your palms into the mat as you draw your shoulder blades back and stretch them. Keep your head in line with your spine making sure to not let it hang.

Stay in this pose for 1 minute.

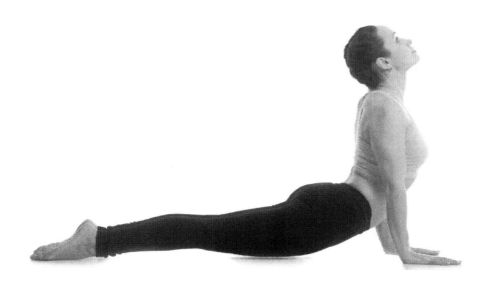

Day 19: Upward Facing Dog

Step 1: Lie in the floor on your stomach and extend your legs out behind you with the tops of your feet pressed against the floor. Move your forearms perpendicular to the floor and place your palms on the floor on either side of you.

Step 2: As you inhale, press your hands into the floor like you're going to do a push up, straighten the arms as your lift your torso and legs off the floor.

Step 3: Push your tailbone down toward your pubic bone and lift your pubic bone to your belly button. Push your shoulder blade back and lift your chest, but don't puff it out. Be careful not to create tension in your lower back. If this happens you can spread your legs wider to relieve the pressure.

Stay in this pose for up to 1 minute. If you feel like you need to counteract the backbend you can do a Child's pose afterward.

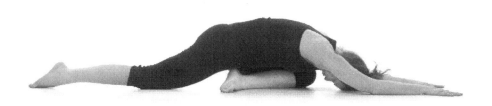

Day 20: Pigeon Pose

Step 1: Get on your hands and knees and bring your right knee up toward your right hand. Angle your right knee slightly and then slide your left leg back as far as you feel comfortable.

Step 2: Be sure to have your hips as square to the floor as possible, otherwise you'll put pressure on your back and this whole pose will be pointless. If you don't feel a deep enough stretch in your right glute then you can slide your right foot forward until you feel like you're in the right position.

Step 3: If you're brand new to this pose you'll probably be most comfortable being up on your hands to keep most of the pressure off your hips. However, if you feel you need more of a stretch you can rest on your forearms or even chest!

As a beginner I recommend staying in this pose for around 30 seconds or whatever is most comfortable to you.

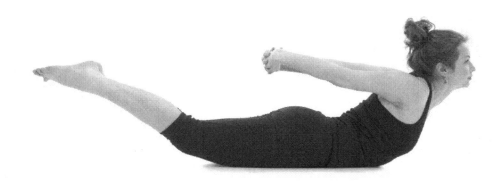

Day 21: Locust Pose

Step 1: For this pose, be sure to either have a soft mat or towel to lie on because otherwise you may be uncomfortable. Start out lying on your stomach with your legs extended behind you and the tops of your feet against the floor. Your arms should be beside you with your palms down.

Step 2: As you inhale, lift your legs and feet, arms and hands, and chest and head off of the floor as high as possible. Keep your shoulders back and engage your back muscles while at the same time relaxing your glute muscles.

Step 3: Be sure to elongate your neck and don't strain while you look forward and breathe in and out.

Stay in this pose for 1 minute and engage your abdominals the entire time.

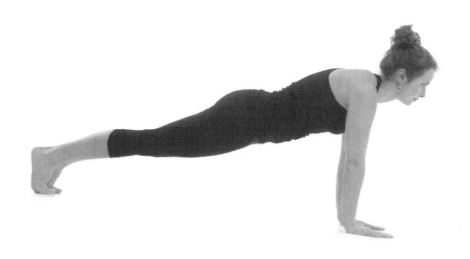

Day 22: Plank Pose

Step 1: Start in Downward Facing Dog. As you inhale bring your torso forward until you have your arms perpendicular to the floor with your shoulders right above your wrists.

Step 2: Be sure to keep your arms straight as you draw your shoulder blades together and broaden your collarbones.

Step 3: Next, engage your core and bring your tailbone toward your heels being sure not to curve your back—you want your spine to be completely straight.

You can stay in this pose for as long as you like or until exhaustion.

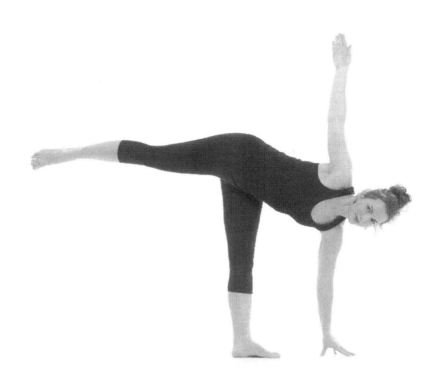

Day 23: Half Moon Pose

Step 1: Start in your Extended Triangle Pose on your right side, then rest your left hand on your left hip. As you inhale slightly bend your right knee and move your left foot forward 6-12 inches. As you do this move your right hand forward at least 12 inches.

Step 2: On the exhale push your right hand and heel into the floor as you straighten the right leg. At the same time, lift your left leg parallel to the floor. Don't hyperextend your right knee—it needs to be aligned forward not inward.

Step 3: Now move your torso the left and keep your left hip slightly forward. As a beginner it would be best to keep your left hand on your hip and your head at a neutral position.

Step 4: Be sure to keep most of your weight on your right leg and if you need to you can help steady yourself with your hand on the floor.

Stay in this position for 1 minute and then repeat on the opposite side.

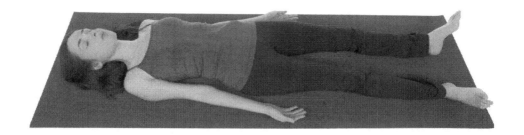

Day 24: Corpse Pose

Step 1: As you lay on your back, focus on lifting the pelvis and sliding the tailbone down to spread out your lower back. Don't arch the back unnaturally and lengthen your legs, resting them hip width apart. Let the feet and legs roll outwards to their natural resting position.

Step 2: Raise your arms and spread your shoulder blades so that they are away from your neck. Rest them at your sides at about a 45-degree angle with your palms up.

Step 3: Visualize and lengthen the neck by placing your chin closer to your chest. Inhale deeply and then exhale as you sink your body into the floor and become quiet and still. Visualize your entire body and it rests and feel your eyes relax and your mouth and face soften.

Use this position as a time for self-reflection and rejuvenation. I suggest doing this pose for at least 5 minutes a day.

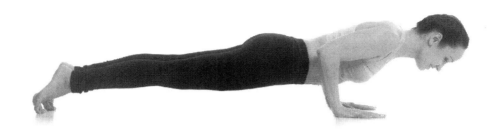

Day 25: Four Limbed Staff

Step 1: Get into Downward Facing Dog and then go into Plank Pose. Keep your shoulder blades firm and your tailbone pulled toward your pubic bone.

Step 2: As you exhale, gently lower the torso and legs just a couple inches parallel to your mat. Be mindful to keep your back properly aligned and straight and keep your pubic bone tucked inward toward the belly button.

Step 3: Make sure to broaden your shoulder blades and keep your elbows close to your sides as you press your fingers into the mat. Left your sternum and head so that you're looking forward.

Stay in this position for up to 30 seconds if you can.

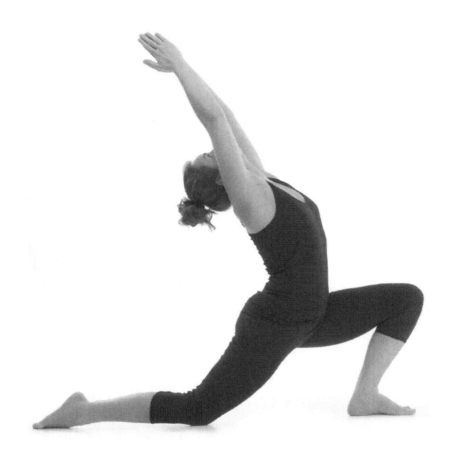

Day 26: Low Lunge

Step 1: Get into Downward Facing Dog. As you exhale bring your right foot up to rest between your hands making sure that the right knee is aligned over the right heel. Next, rest your left knee on the floor and slide it back until you feel a slight stretch in your thigh and groin area. Once you feel the stretch you can rest the top of your left foot on the floor.

Step 2: As you inhale, bring your torso up and in a sweeping motion bring your arms to the sides, perpendicular to the floor. Be sure to keep your chest lifted and your shoulders pressed back.

Step 3: Bring your head up and move your pinkie fingers up to the ceiling. Hold here for a minute and then exhale moving your torso back to your right bringing your hands to the floor and your left toes under. As you exhale again, bring your left knee forward and get back into Downward Facing Dog.

Repeat this pose for the opposite side.

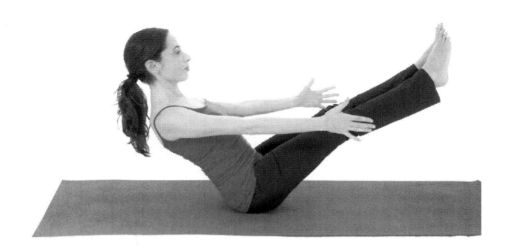

Day 27: Boat Pose

Step 1: In a sitting position put your knees and feet together with your knees bent. Hold the backs of your knees and focus on lengthening the spine as you lean back slightly making sure not to fold over as you find the edge of your butt bones.

Step 2: Stare straight ahead and as you inhale bring your feet a couple inches off the ground, balancing on your butt, breathing in and out as you find your balance.

Step 3: Stay tall as you gently raise your heels to knee level, keeping your knees bent. If you can complete this easily and you're comfortable then let go of your legs and bring your arms forward as you keep chest broad. If you still feel good and steady you can raise your legs at a diagonal in the air in front of you taking care not to round your back.

Stay in this position for as long as you can, but at least 30 seconds.

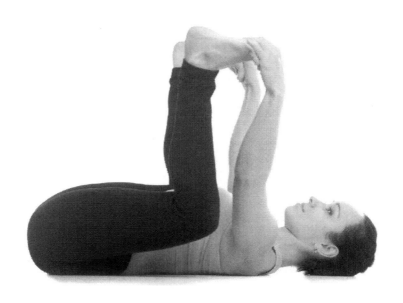

Day 28: Happy Baby Pose

Step 1: Lie on the floor on your back. As you exhale, bring your knees into your stomach.

Step 2: On an inhale, grab the outside of both feet and open your knees up a little wider than the width of your torso. Pull your feet up towards your armpits.

Step 3: Bring both ankles directly over your knees, making your shins perpendicular to the floor as you flex through your heels. Gently push up with your feet while at the same time pulling your hands down to create a resistant stretch.

Stay in this pose as long as you're comfortable or 1 minute.

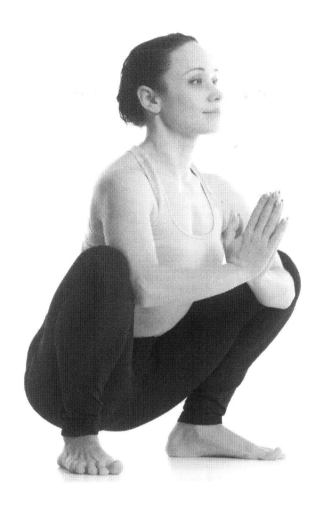

Day 29: Garland Pose

Step 1: Get into a squatting position with your feet as close as you can get them to each other, keeping your heels flat on the floor.

Step 2: Make sure your thighs are a little wider than the width of your torso and as you exhale, lean forward to fit comfortably between your thighs.

Step 3: Bring your elbows to the inside of your knees and place your palms together in prayer position being mindful of keeping your torso upright and not slouching.

Stay in this position for up to 1 minute.

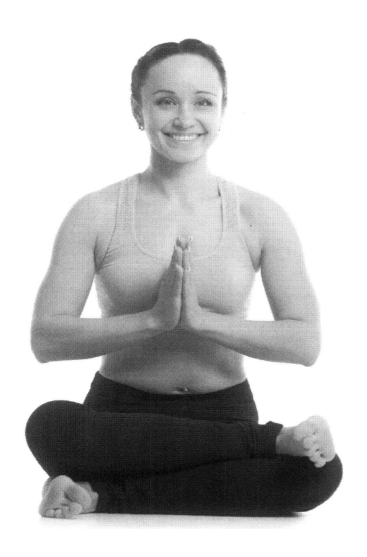

Day 30: Fire Log Pose

Step 1: First, sit down on your mat and bend your knees out in front of you so that your feet are flat on the floor and your palms are resting on the floor behind you.

Step 2: Lean back and cross your right ankle over the left knee keeping the right foot flexed and away from the knee until you feel a stretch in the right hip.

Step 3: Slowly walk your left foot back to the right as you move your hands forward to sit up straight and stack the legs. Next, line your right foot over the left knee and then the right knee over the left ankle. The goal is to make the shins be parallel.

Step 4: If you want more of a stretch you can place your hands out in front of you and lean forward, otherwise just stay in the upright position.

Stay here for up to 1 minute then release.

Chapter 7: Achieving Inner Peace Through Yoga

Is it Really Possible?

By now you should be caught up on all the basics of yoga and you may even consider yourself more intermediate than novice at this point. But before you move on to practicing more advanced moves and techniques I just want to share with you what yoga means to me and why it's more than just how flexible and bendy you are.

It's completely okay, if in the beginning, your biggest concern is how flexible you can get or simply becoming more toned. I was exactly that way when I first started yoga; I'll admit that it was mostly for vanity purposes.

As time has passed, though, and I've delved deeper into my practice yoga has become so much more than just a form of exercise to me—it has become my livelihood. This might sound a little extreme, but trust me when I say that yoga has completely transformed my mindset and personality and that I wouldn't be who I am today without it.

Over the years something just clicked inside of me—my reasons for practicing yoga slowly changed and the things that once motivated me to do it (like the challenge of a new pose) got replaced by an inner *need* for my "me time." I needed a time to reflect and be quiet in my mind and yoga became that outlet.

I know that not everyone is into the spiritual or religious side of things and I get that. If I'm being honest, when I first started practicing yoga I didn't really feel all that spiritual and I sure as heck wasn't religious. Why am I telling you this? Because I want you to know that if you give yoga a chance it might just change your life. You will experience more happiness and inner peace and tranquility than you ever even knew was possible.

It all might sound too good to be true and I'm definitely not saying all of this to try and put yoga up on some sort of pedestal. I love it and I hope that you love it, too, but I realize that it's not going to be the same experience for everyone. And personally I think that that's 100% okay.

If we all just embrace *our* own version of yoga—whatever that may be—and use our time in practice to become the best versions of ourselves that we possibly can I think the world would be a much better place and we'd all find the everlasting happiness and tranquility we've all been searching for all along.

Conclusion

So you've made it to the end of this crazy rollercoaster of a book! I feel like a proud parent watching her child walk across the stage at graduation. But really, though, congratulations on completing *Yoga For Beginners*.

If you've made it the full 30 Days—how does it feel? Are you practicing a little each day, working to become better at each pose? Or maybe you've even moved on and taken a class or tried some more challenging poses?

Either way, you should feel proud of yourself for sticking through and reaching the end—even if that doesn't mean you're "done" with all the poses in the book. And it's okay if you feel slightly overwhelmed by all that you've just read and you haven't even started—I get it.

My only request from you is this: please don't make the mistake of *never starting*. Give yoga a chance to change your life and your mindset. I promise you won't regret it!

Love and light,
Olivia

Printed in Great Britain
by Amazon